Keto Diet

Ketogenic Diet guide for beginners to lose weight and burn body-fat fast

Simon Donovan

Table of Contents

Introduction

The Paleo Diet. The Atkins Diet. The South Beach Diet...What do all these diets have in common?

If you're like most people who tried diets in the past, you're probably well-aware of these diets. Did you know that they have a common thread running through them? That's right, they all use ketosis to produce results.

Ketosis may sound scary. It may sound like it refers to some sort of wasting disease or some sort of nasty open sores, but the reality is actually quite positive. Ketosis is the process where your body burns your fat stores for energy. This is quite different from how your body normally gets energy. Normally, your body gets its energy in the form of sugar in your blood stream.

There are three types of food: "Go," "Grow," and "Glow" foods

Glow foods give you nutrients and vitamins that you need for optimal health. Grow foods involve protein. Protein is required for tissue synthesis. You need protein to grow your muscle mass. Go foods, other hand, give you energy. These are foods that are high in starch, sugar, and carbohydrates.

With ketosis, your focus is to eat more foods that help you grow and reduce Go foods. The big difference between the Paleo, Atkins, and South Beach diets is the specific spin they put on the ketogenic process. They all share ketosis, but they have varying levels of grains, sugar, carbs, and daily inputs. They also vary based upon the types of animal protein they allow. In short, they impose varying rules that dictate the amount and kind of foods you eat.

This book spells out a purely Ketogenic Diet. My focus is on how to trigger ketosis as efficiently as possible. Before I begin, I'd like to share my personal story.

I've always struggled with my weight ever since high school. It seems that no matter what diet I tried, I could not get rid of the extra 50 pounds I was saddled with. Now, don't get me wrong. I would try diet after diet and supplement after supplement, and they would work. I can't deny that for a certain amount of time, I will lose weight. Maybe it's 10 pounds here, 20 pounds there.

What's really frustrating about this whole process is that eventually my appetite would get the better of me and I would regain all the weight that I lost. The secret to successful dieting is not losing weight. Most diets work on some level or other. They will help you lose pounds here and there, but that's not your objective is to lose weight and keep it off.

In personal situation, the Keto Diet is the only diet that helped me get rid of the 50 pounds that I was lugging around since high school. The best part is that I kept it off. I can say with a lot of certainty that it's gone for good. My secret? The Keto Diet that you will learn throughout this book.

Chapter 1: The Key To ANY Diet Success

Before I dive into the mechanics of the Keto Diet, I just want to make something clear: If you don't have the right mindset, you will fail! You need to wrap your mind around this. A lot of people think that losing weight is just something that you experience physically. Worse, many people think that weight loss is something that's fully external to them. If this is your mindset, chances are quite high you will fail. Here are the reasons why.

Diet versus lifestyle

People who are able to lose weight on a permanent basis do not engage in diets. Instead, they modify their lifestyles. This is crucial because people on diets eventually regain all the weight that they have lost. To make things worse, they actually end up gaining more weight than they lost in the first place. You have to resolve to change your lifestyle. This is the only way to permanent weight loss.

Lifestyle change is quite difficult for many people not because it's physically hard, but because it requires a change in mindset. It's easy to make physical changes. I mean, I can change clothes, or I can change my choices of shoes. What's more difficult is changing the way I think. This is precisely what's needed for permanent weight loss.

The problem with typical weight-loss programs is that they aren't permanent. They focus on an external source. Diet book after diet book hype up an external way to lose weight. They say that if you just eat this type of supplement, you will lose weight. They say that if you follow a certain eating routine and time it right, you will lose weight. If you keep things at an external level, you won't achieve permanent results. This piece of advice also applies to the contents of this book.

You can read this book backwards and forwards, and truly absorb its information, but if you don't change your mindset, it's not going to lead to permanent results. Put simply, if you change your mindset, the weight loss this book enables you to attain will be permanent.

Key mindset requirements

There are certain fundamental things that you need to believe for this book to truly work for you. You can follow the tips outlined throughout this book on an item by item basis and get results. That's not the problem. The problem is making sure that whatever weight-loss results you get become permanent. The way to do this is to believe in certain things. I'm going to lay out certain beliefs that you really need to internalize, otherwise this book will only produce temporary relief from your struggle with your weight.

Believe it is possible to lose weight permanently

The first thing that I need you to believe is that it's possible to lose weight permanently. I know you're probably skeptical at this point in time. After all, you are probably a veteran of many different weight-loss programs.

You've tried many different diet books. All of them make the same claim. All of them have slick packaging. You've heard all sorts of weight-loss terms thrown at you. You're probably aware of all sorts of weight-loss seminars and programs. It's easy to get jaded. It's easy to look at your frustrations at attaining permanent weight loss.

Well, I'm telling you, if you do not believe that it's possible to lose weight permanently, then it won't be possible. It really is that simple. You have to open your mind to the possibility that you can say good-bye to that nasty spare tire around your midsection. As the old saying goes, "For you to achieve, you must first believe." If you want to change your personal reality permanently, you must first believe that it is possible to achieve permanent change.

Your comfort and mood doesn't have to come from food

A lot of people who struggle with their weight are frustrated in their weight-loss efforts because they have an unhealthy relationship with food. They eat primarily because of emotional triggers and emotional rewards. It's very easy to see how this can lead to bad results. If you feel bad about your self-image and you think you don't look all that good or you're too fat, you are looking for comfort, and you look at food like snacks or chocolate cakes as sources of reassurance and comfort. You're just making things much worse for yourself.

The more you eat, the more weight you pack on. When you look at the mirror, you feel worse about yourself and this triggers another round of eating. Do you see where this is all headed? Do you see how the process of comfort eating defeats your efforts to lose weight permanently?

Stop looking at food as a source of comfort. Your source of comfort must come from within. It must not come from somebody else. It must not come from food that lies outside of yourself. It must come from you. You must validate yourself. You have to be more proactive in setting or managing your moods from within, instead of constantly being triggered by external stimuli like food or other people.

Your circumstances don't determine your mood, your values do

I've already started to move your source of mood from external sources to internal sources with my previous tip. With this tip, we're going to improve further on that point. Your circumstances must never determine your mood. Instead of constantly reacting to what's going on around you, focus more on what your values are and focus more on the things that provide you with confidence. In other words, stop reacting and start acting proactively.

When your mood is set by your values, it doesn't really matter what's going on around you, what people are saying, and what kind of food you're tempted by. Your values will prevail. You will know the proper way to respond and the proper outcome to shoot for. When you let your inner values dictate your response to the outside world, you win. It really is that simple.

Unfortunately, people who have problems with self-control or self-discipline and comfort eating, base their mood on their surroundings. If certain people say certain things, they get into a certain mood. If they see certain foods, they get into a certain mood. You have to take your emotional triggers from the external world and center them instead on internal values. The best part of all of this is that you get to choose, which values you proactively link with certain moods.

Of course, this process doesn't happen overnight. In many cases, this is a purely intellectual exercise at first but the more you practice this, the stronger you become internally.

Eventually, you would reach a point where external triggers no longer set you off. You gain a tremendous amount of personal control because it will be your values that are driving your moods and your choices.

Your external reality is just a reflection of your inner reality

The next time you look in the mirror, take a long hard look at what you look like. Everything about you, from how much you weigh to the clothes you choose, to your haircut, is a reflection of your inner values. Everything that you see is just a reflection of what's going on within you. It's really important to fully understand this because if the external is a reflection of the internal, you have a tremendous amount of power. Why? You are always in control of the things that you choose to think about.

If what you think about has a direct impact on your external reality, then you have a lot of control. You actually have a lot more power of your life than you give yourself credit for. It all boils down to consciously and deliberately thinking of certain things instead of other things.

When you think the way you normally do, it produces predictable results, obviously since you're trying to lose weight, it's not producing the kind of results that you're happy with. You can change all of this by simply changing the way you think. Change your internal reality and change how you perceive yourself on the inside, ultimately this would have a profound effect of what you look like on the outside.

The more you exercise self-control, the stronger it becomes

Think of your self-control as a muscle. Body builders weren't born with that physique. Usually, they were born with chicken chests and thin arms. They got that big because they exercised their muscles. The same applies to your self-control or any other personal trait. The more you challenge it and the more you use it, the stronger your self-control becomes. The more you resist that chocolate cake in the fridge, the easier it would be for you to resist it in the future.

You have to remember that the reverse is also true. The more you give in to temptation, the weaker your self-control becomes. It just becomes easier and easier for you to give in. It becomes easier and easier for you to overeat. Eventually, you would lose, for all practice purposes, the self-control that you need to keep your weight in check.

Unlock the power of momentum

The hardest part in any kind of project is starting. This should not be a surprise. After all, you haven't done that thing before. There's a lot of uncertainty. Most people are scared of change. You don't know what to expect. However, the moment you try something, the easier it is to keep trying again. The moment you do something, the easier it is to do that thing again.

Let's put it this way, when a rocket is sent into outer space, most of that rocket's fuel are used up in the first few minutes. Why? You need a tremendous amount of fuel to escape the Earth's gravity. However, once the rocket reaches a certain point, it takes less energy to go much farther into space. Ultimately, the rocket will reach a point that it doesn't take much energy at all to go at an extremely fast speed. The reason is simple. It's all about initial inertia and gravity.

By the same token, if you are trying to adopt a healthier lifestyle of eat certain foods that will trigger ketosis, your body will put up a fight. It's harder to get started because you don't know what to expect because you haven't done it before.

The good news is that the longer you stick with the Keto Diet that I will teach you, the easier it would be for you to make the right food choices. Eventually, it becomes a habit, and you are able to achieve greater and greater results. Ultimately, becomes a part of your lifestyle, and you stop looking at it as a diet. It's not something that you do every once in a while. It becomes a part of who you are.

The bottom line

The bottom line with any kind of diet success is to stop looking at symptoms. You can poke at the symptoms all you want, but unless you address the root causes, you're not going to make any permanently progress. This applies to all areas of your life. We're not just talking about losing weight. We're also talking about building better relationships and establishing more discipline, so you can achieve a higher degree of power. You cannot just poke at the symptoms. You also have to knock out the cause.

The cause of most weight problems is mindset. There are many people who have metabolic and medical issues that prevent them from losing weight on a permanent basis. I'm not talking about those individuals. If you are like most other people, the main reason why your weight-loss efforts don't yield permanent results is because your mindset. Stop looking at losing weight as a technical issue and look at it as a mindset issue. Adopt the mindsets I've outlined above, and you will explode your chances of saying good-bye permanently to your extra weight.

Chapter 2: Keto or Ketogenic Diet basics

The origin of the Ketogenic Diet is actually quite ancient. Even in the days of the Ancient Greeks, there is classical medical literature that point to fasting as a means to cut down on epileptic seizures. This involves simply stopping eating. By the late 1800s, physicians modified classical anti-epilepsy fasting diets to cut down on a specific category of food: Starchy foods.

Doctors in the 1800s noticed that when they took out grains and carb-rich items from the diets of their patients, this drastically reduced the frequency of their epileptic fits. There was quite a bit of progress made using dietary treatments for epilepsy until the dawn of modern anti-seizure meditations in the 1920s. Since meditation provided much faster relief to seizures, most medical practitioners abandoned carb-free to control epilepsy.

Interestingly enough, in the medical literature of the late 1800s all the way up to the 1940s, one of the most common "side effects" of the carb-free diet is persistent weight loss. Fast-forward to our modern age, there's been no shortage of Ketogenic Diets whether we're talking about the Atkins Diet or South Beach Diet. What do they have in common? All of them emphasize lower carbohydrate intake while increasing protein and fat.

One of the most popular diets currently is the Paleo Diet. This diet simulates the food choices of our distant ancestors. Supposedly, by eating very minimal grains, skipping out or reducing on dairy, and loading up on meat will not only be healthier for you but can also help you lose weight permanently.

The assumption behind the Paleo Diet is that modern physiology hasn't fully evolved enough to fit our modern grain-based diet. Similarly, there's a heavy emphasis on organic food in a lot of the variants of the Paleo Diet out there. The focus here is to try to simulate the diet of cavemen and prehistoric man because this is supposedly healthier.

The reason why these contemporary low-carb high protein diets work is quite simple actually. They use ketosis. In this chapter, I'm going to spell out the ketosis process and how ketogenic weight loss works.

The ketosis process

Your body has only three sources of energy. It can burn the sugar found in your blood stream. It can free up the calories stored in your fat tissue by burning fat, and finally it can get calories by burning up your muscle mass.

Typically, most people get their energy source from the sugar that they eat every single day. This, of course, is not sugar in a highly-refined form. Most people get their sugar in the form of carbohydrates or starchy foods like bread, pasta, rice, and other grain-based foods. Rarely do people just eat pure sugar. Still, your body breaks down carbohydrates into a form of sugar that it can then metabolize into energy.

How ketogenic weight loss works

Before I get into ketogenic weight loss, let me devote some time to how weight loss normally works. Your body only loses weight in one of three ways. First, you can cut down the amount of calories you eat every day. When you do this, your body still burns calories at its previous rate. This creates a net negative calorie state where your body needs more calories than the calories that you're taking in.

Your body has to look for those "missing" calories. It first burns up the sugar in your blood stream. Once this is gone, your body then looks at your stored fat and burns that for calories. Depending on how you eat and your overall lifestyle, your body might also simultaneously burn fat and muscle for calories. If you eat in a ketogenic way, your body burns fat first before breaking down your muscle mass for energy.

The other scenario involves eating the same amount of calories per day, but increasing the level of physical activity you engage in. This is just a fancy way to say exercising more or moving around more. Maybe you've made it a habit to park very far from the places that you visit. This forces you to walk longer distances. Maybe you've adopted the habit of taking the stairs instead of riding the elevator.

However you decide to do it, simply moving around more increases the calorie requirement of your body, and this triggers a net negative calorie state if you eat the same calories as before, when this happens the same process that I've described above plays out. Your body will look for those "missing" calories, and you end up losing weight.

Another way you can boost your body's passive calorie burn rate is to lift weights or do resistance exercises. These build up your muscle mass due to microscopic tears. Not only do bigger muscles need more calories to maintain, repairing the micro tears from your weight training boosts your body's calorie requirements even further.

The third approach to weight loss is a combination of eating less and moving around more. This is actually the most optimal way to lose weight because you drastically increase the net negative calorie state your body is in. Your body's calorie requirement increases tremendously and it burns more sugar, fat, or muscle to make up for the calories it's no longer taking in.

The benefits of the Ketogenic Diet

A Ketogenic Diet uses ketosis for its calorie requirements. By reducing your carbohydrate or sugar intake on a prolonged basis, your body is forced to turn to your fat stores for energy. This is a very efficient way to lose weight because once you achieve ketosis, your body starts burning fat.

Since your body is no longer using blood sugar to determine hunger cycles, your body's cells are more sensitive to insulin. This helps prevent the onset of diabetes. You also feel less hungry because your body is no longer using blood sugar levels to detect hunger. Your body is burning fat at an even rate, and this has the effect of smoothing out your hunger cycles. Don't get me wrong, you will still feel hungry at certain parts during the day, but they're not as extreme as when you eat a lot of high glycemic index foods like rice, white bread, and pasta.

This all leads to lower overall hunger levels. You'll feel fuller longer, and you tend to eat less. Since you're eating less, you will achieve a net negative calorie state more frequently, and this leads to further weight loss.

Eventually, your new diet recalibrates your hunger cycle, and you are able to remain at a certain amount of calorie intake every day, and you maintain your lower weight.

Chapter 3: Easy Ketogenic Diet Guidelines

As I've mentioned in the introduction, the Ketogenic Diet is actually all over the place. It just has many different variations. For a pure Keto Diet, you need to get a clear understanding of fat. Fat is crucial for triggering ketosis. If you eat a certain amount and a certain range of fat types, you jump-start the ketosis process. Unfortunately, a lot of people still think that all fat is bad for you. I really can't say I blame them because for the longest time, the U.S. Department of Health had guidelines that said all cholesterol is bad and all fat is bad, but it turns out that this was based on a bad reading and interpretation of dietary scientific literature.

To ensure optimal ketosis, you need to adopt the following advice.

Eat more fat, modern protein, and reduce carbohydrates as much as possible

As much as possible, try to keep your daily carb intake below 100 grams. For protein intake, one powerful formula suggested by Volek and Phinney uses a minimum and maximum threshold. Take your weight (in pounds) and multiply it by .6. The resulting figure is the minimum grams of protein you should eat daily. To find maximum protein intake, take your weight and multiply by 1. Example: If I weigh 200 pounds, the minimum amount of protein I should eat daily is 120 grams while the maximum is 200 grams.

Myth busted: Not all fat is bad for you

To trigger ketosis, fat is required. The problem is that it's too easy to just rush to animal-based fat. This can cause serious issues because animal-based fat is loaded with cholesterol and is polysaturated fat. If you load up on too much of this type of fat, it can cause more problems than it solves. It can cause hardening of arteries and hypertension. High animal fat diets have also been linked to increased chances of developing diabetes.

The good news is that there are certain types of fat out there that is great for you. These are medium chain fats. Among all these medium chain fats, coconut oil stands out really well. If you load up on coconut oil, this gives your body the fat that it needs to start the ketosis process. It starts burning up the coconut oil you ingested and it starts burning up your stored fat as your body gets used to using fat for its primary source of energy. Use medium chain fats like coconut oil to get the ketosis process going.

After you have determined your maximum carbohydrate and protein intake, the rest of your calories will come from healthy oils. Because they are so calorie dense, oil and fats take care of your cravings and you feel fuller longer.

What oils should you eat?

Try to stick to vegetable-based oils like oils sources from coconuts, olives, avocados, macadamias, red palms, and palms. For added flavor and variety, you can try out nut-based oils but keep them to a low level. Animal-based fats are allowed but, due to the health concerns raised above, keep your intake to a moderate amount. Try low to moderate amounts of pork lard, duck fat, beef fat or tallow.

What foods should you load up on?

Now that you're eating more oil to get the ketosis process going, you also need to watch what categories of food to eat. You need to get rid of carbohydrates as much as possible or outright eliminate grains like rice, wheat, corn and any food items that have high-starch content from your diet. Instead, load up on lean meat proteins. These can take the form of chicken breast or some cuts of pork. Goat meat is particularly lean. Any cut of meat with its fat trimmed off is good for a high-protein diet. Of course, as much as possible, you should focus on the leanest types and cuts of meats.

If you're looking for flavorful, calorie-dense, protein-packed treats, try organ meats. They are packed tight with nutrients. Prepared right, organ meats can be very tasty.

Quick warning about too much meat in your diet

While you should load up on protein, make sure you stay within your minimum and maximum daily intake range. Too much protein in your diet actually slows down the ketosis process.

Shellfish and seafood

Shellfish and seafood are packed with protein, fat, and flavor. If you have access to affordable seafood, load up on it. Try shellfish, abalone, clams crab, lobster, mussels, oysters, shrimp, scallops, and squid.

Personally, I prefer fish and lean chicken breast. Fish is especially a good addition to your diet because in addition to the lean protein that they pack, deep-sea fish also a high level of Omega 3. Omega 3 is great for your brain, heart health, and overall health. Try to buy mostly wild caught fish instead of farmed fish. Farmed fish can accumulate toxins and heavy metals.

What about Fruit?

As a rule of thumb, you should avoid most fruits due to their carb content. If you need to eat fruit try eating only small amounts of berries. This restriction on fruit applies to dried fruits as well since their sugar content is concentrated by the drying process

What about legumes like peanuts and soy/tofu?

Legumes are banned in the ketogenic diet due to their carb content and ketosis-retarding qualities

Nuts in your Ketogenic meal plans

Nuts are okay but in moderation due to their carb content.

Ketogenic strategy

When starting your diet, load up on the oils and gradually increase the amount of protein in your diet. Start displacing the grains in your diet. It's a good idea to start this out gradually. You don't want a shock and awe approach because your system gets so shaken up that it instinctively fights back. It might not fight back immediately, but it will start to push back gradually. Eventually, you go back to your old eating patterns.

It's much better to displace the foods that you were eating before by loading up on protein and then dialing back on the amount of carbohydrates you eat. Once your body starts losing ketones for hunger signals instead of sugar, it becomes much easier to eliminate grains and starchy foods outright.

Optional foods

While you should load up on protein and reduce carbohydrates, there are certain plant-based foods you should eat more of. I'm talking about high-fiber foods like flax seed. Flax seed is loaded with omega fatty acids and fiber. Fiber is important because it cleans out your gastrointestinal tract, and it helps you feel fuller for a longer time.

When you have a lot of dietary fiber in your system, it swells up when it gets in contact with the water in your stomach, and you end up feeling fuller. Since you feel fuller longer, you tend to eat less, and this reduces your overall calorie intake. This then, of course, leads to even more weight loss. Eventually, once high-fiber components are incorporated in your diet, and your system gets used to it, your lower weight stabilizes.

Chapter 4 : Sugar: White, Pure, Deadly

As I've mentioned previously, there are ketogenic foods, such as high-protein foods and certain types of fat, that help spurs the ketosis process. There is also one class of food that is its antithesis. This is the anti-ketogenic compound of sugar. Starchy foods, when purified, take the form of sugar. Sugar is bad news, seriously. Purified sugar is the one food item that you must absolutely avoid if you want to lose weight through ketosis. If there is any one food that is just completely forbidden, it is purified sugar. Check below for the reasons why.

The dangers of sugar

Whether you drink sugar in the form of soda, or you eat it in the form of starchy foods like pasta and rice. Sugar packs a wide range of health risks. First, too much sugar in your blood stream eventually leads to insulin resistance. This means that you have to eat more sugar so just enough sugar could get into your cells. Since sugar in the blood stream is biochemically toxic, it doesn't take a genius to see why this can lead to chronic health problems like diabetes and certain types of cancer.

Your pancreas goes through a tremendous amount of pressure when there is too much sugar in your blood stream, and eventually you can develop pancreatitis or pancreatic cancer. Pancreatic cancer is almost a death sentence. Its morbidity rate, as far as cancers go, is extremely high. Another reason why sugar is bad for you is that it simply primes your body for maximizing calorie intake. When you get hungry, it takes a lot more food to get rid of the hunger signals. Your body simply becomes dependent on detecting blood sugar to determine whether it's hungry.

If your blood sugar is artificially elevated for a long period of time, then your body's whole hunger signal system is thrown off track. Keep this up for a long enough period of time and your body's hunger signal system is thrown off track pretty much permanently. You end up pretty much hungry for most of the time. This boosts your overall calorie intake.

Finally, if you eat a lot of sugar, whether in the form of ingredients, starch, or purified sugar, whatever diet you go on is eventually going to be a yoyo diet. You're not going to achieve permanent weight loss. Your body will still look at your blood-sugar level to determine hunger, and you're going to be stuck on a weight-loss treadmill. You lose weight when you diet then you gain it all back plus a few more pounds, you then go on another diet, and you lose some weight, and you then gain back the weight. It just goes on and on because sugar is still in the picture.

The most dangerous thing about sugar

As troubling as the dangers I've mentioned above are, what's really alarming about sugar is the fact that it's everywhere. Thanks to high-fructose corn syrup, sugar is pretty much everywhere. In the United States, sugar can be found in anything from "high-fiber" cookies to toothpaste and all points in between. High-fructose corn syrup is so cheap and so plentiful that it's the preferred choice of many food manufacturers for a cheap sweetening agent. Not surprisingly, sugar can be found everywhere and its dangers are often disguised.

Stop drinking your calories!

One of the most basic ways you can lose weight is to simply stop drinking your calories. That's right, by simply skipping soda drinks that are sweetened by high-fructose corn syrup, you can start losing weight. By switching to water, you knock off a tremendous amount of carb-based calories off your daily eating schedule. If you're looking for a quick and easy start to a Ketogenic Diet, start with knocking sugar-sweetened soda drinks off the menu.

Don't get tricked by sugar-free drinks

It's very tempting to switch from regular soda to sugar-free soda. After all, these sugar-free drinks are advertised as being completely free of sugar. Don't fall for the advertising hype. While it is true that these drinks do not pack any calories because they don't have sugar, they are also loaded with metabolism-altering compounds. They are so loaded with chemicals that they can wreak havoc with your metabolism. You may not be drinking any sugar with these drinks, but they might be slowing down the rate at which your body burns calories or processes fat into calories.

Chapter 5 : Rounding Out Your Ketogenic Diet

One of the most common myths about Ketogenic Diets is that they are just for meat-eaters. This is absolutely not true. You can be on a Ketogenic Diet and be a vegetarian, no joke. In fact, a well-rounded Ketogenic Diet involves vegetables. If you want to be healthier while losing weight permanently, you need to include veggies and high-fiber components into your diet. Here are just some recommendations.

Dark-green leafy vegetables

As a rule of thumb, if you're going to be adding salads or roughage to your meal plans, stick to dark green leafy vegetables like kale, rocket arugula, lettuce, and leeks. You should also try chard.

Broccoli and other protein-heavy veggies

Did you know that there are many vegetables that are loaded with protein? I'm not talking about peanuts and nuts in general. You should keep these to a minimum. Instead, focus on veggies like broccoli. In fact, you can come close to getting all your protein needs with just one serving of broccoli.

Loading up on fiber the right way

As I've mentioned previously, you should load up on fiber. Not only does fiber make you feel fuller much longer, it also can help you clean out your gut efficiently and quickly. A well functioning gastrointestinal tract leads to better overall health. It's also important to match up the heavy amount of protein in your diet with vegetables, which contains a decent amount of fiber.

If you load up on a moderate of meat and there's not enough fiber, your gastrointestinal tract might be vulnerable to certain types of cancer. Loading up on veggies with decent or high-levels of fiber helps ensure a clean gastrointestinal tract, and you also get the added advantage of antioxidants, nutrients, and vitamins that protein-heavy vegetables with decent fiber content bring to the table.

Here is a supplemental list of vegetables you should consider adding to your meal plan

Artichokes
Asparagus
Bell Peppers
Brussels Sprouts
Cabbage
Carrots
Cauliflower
Celery
Chives
Garlic
Mushrooms
Mustard Greens
Okra
Onions
Parsley
Peppers
Pumpkin
Seaweed
Shallots
Tomatoes
Turnip Greens

Watercress
Zucchini

A final word about Veggies

Stick to the list above. Avoid starchy root crops as much as possible.

Chapter 6: Ketogenic Lifestyle Tips

As I've mentioned previously, if you want to lose weight permanently, you have to modify your lifestyle. You can't just go from diet to diet. When adopting the Ketogenic Diet tips included in this book, you may also want to make the following changes to your lifestyle.

Wake up early

When you wake up early, your body's metabolic system kicks into gear. Your internal body processes start burning calories much sooner than usual. This can help your body burn up calories much more efficiently and much more cleanly. Besides the metabolic benefits, waking up early also helps you increase the amount of willpower you have. Assuming that you had a full night's sleep, waking up early enables you to enjoy a much higher amount of willpower and this can pay off tremendously when you're faced with tempting food choices.

Discipline is crucial in sticking to a diet. If you are trying to change your lifestyle, so you weigh less, and you eat healthier, you need to make the right decisions as far as food choices go on a consistent basis. This is impossible to do unless you have a high enough level of willpower. You have to consistently choose ketogenic foods over sugary snacks, foods with high-levels to the wrong kind of fat, and starchy foods. In many cases, it would feel that your whole body is craving for something sweet. Of course, the more you resist your body's cravings, the more willpower you will need.

Waking up early and getting a full night's sleep will give you the amount of willpower you require to constantly make the right decisions. The good news is the more you pick the right foods, the higher the likelihood that this will become a habit. However, until you develop healthier eating habits, you need a large amount of willpower.

Time your meals properly

Your body burns more calories in the early to middle part during the day compared to the later part of the day. As you get closer to evenings, your body starts to slow down in terms of the rate at which it burns calories. By simply choosing to eat the bulk of your daily calorie intake before 3:00 PM, you increase the likelihood that you will store less fat. This should not come as a surprise. You are simply scheduling your calorie intake to the parts to the day where your body burns the most calories.

By simply choosing not to eat dinner, you drastically improve the likelihood that you would lose weight. This of course takes quite a bit of willpower. If you are used to eating three square meals a day with the biggest meal being dinner, your body is going to put up quite a fight. This is quite a drastic change. Still, by slowly dialing down on the amount of food you eat for dinner, you increase the likelihood that a ketogenic lifestyle will help you lose weight permanently. In fact, I would suggest that you skip dinner entirely and move the bulk of your calorie intake to breakfast or lunch.

Drink more water if you're hungry

By loading up on water when you're hungry, you interrupt your hunger signals because water bulks up your gastrointestinal tract and by drinking more water, there are more fluids to bulk up the fiber in your system. Drinking water also distributes biochemical compounds throughout your system, and this leads to higher levels of satiety. By simply loading up on water when you feel hungry, you decrease your hunger pangs, and this can lead to better weight loss.

Conclusion

Weight loss is primarily mental, not physical. Weight loss on a physical level is actually quite simple. It's a simple matter of calories in, calories out. When you reduce the amount of calories you eat every day, you trigger a net negative calorie state which forces your body to burn up fat. You can also work on the other side of the equation by increasing the amount of calories you burn while keeping the amount of calories you eat at the same level.

Regardless of how you do it, a net negative calorie state is required for people to lose weight. The good news is that by simply choosing different foods to eat, you can trigger this negative calorie state. Best of all, you can train your body to burn up your fat stores, so you look leaner, more muscular, and more toned.

This book highlights key eating strategies that would make ketosis more likely, and also fine-tune and enhance the results that you get. Most importantly, you have to have the right mindset in order for ketosis to produce optimal weight-loss benefits for you over the long term. I wish you nothing but the best in your weight-loss efforts.

www.ingramcontent.com/pod-product-compliance
Lightning Source LLC
Chambersburg PA
CBHW062032280526
45787CB00005B/2293